GLUTEN FREE DIET

A beginners guide to prepare a gluten free diet

Dr Rowan Theo

Table of Contents

CHAPTER ONE 3

The Gluten-Free Diet:...............3

CHAPTER TWO 11

Celiac Disease 11

CHAPTER THREE 24

Health Benefits of a Gluten-Free Diet.....................................24

CHAPTER FOUR 31

Negative Effects.......................31

CHAPTER FIVE......................39

Gluten-Free Menu 39

THE END...................................49

CHAPTER ONE

The Gluten-Free Diet: A Beginner's Guide With Meal Plan

A gluten-unfastened weight loss program includes except for meals that comprise the protein gluten, along with wheat, rye and barley.

Most research on gluten-unfastened diets had been achieved on human beings with celiac sickness, however there may be any other situation known as gluten sensitivity that still reasons troubles with gluten.

If you're illiberal to gluten, you then definately want to keep away from it absolutely. If now no longer, you'll enjoy excessive soreness and unfavorable fitness results.

Here is a entire manual to the gluten-unfastened weight loss program, along with a scrumptious pattern menu. But first, allows begin with the basics.

What Is Gluten?

Gluten is a own circle of relatives of proteins located in wheat, barley, rye and spelt.

Its call comes from the Latin phrase for "glue," because it offers flour a sticky consistency whilst blended with water.

This glue-like assets facilitates gluten create a sticky community that offers bread the cap potential to upward push whilst baked. It additionally offers bread a chewy and gratifying texture.

Unfortunately, many human beings sense uncomfortable after ingesting meals that comprise gluten. The maximum excessive response is known as celiac sickness.

Celiac sickness is an autoimmune ailment wherein the frame mistakenly harms itself. Celiac sickness influences as much as 1%

of the populace and may harm the intestines.

If ingesting gluten makes you sense uncomfortable, it's quality to inform your physician.

These are the maximum common approaches to check for celiac sickness .

• Blood check. A blood check will search for antibodies that incorrectly have interaction with the gluten protein. The maximum common check is a tTG-IgA check.

• Biopsy out of your small gut. People with a nice blood check will in all likelihood want to have a biopsy. This is a procedure wherein a small tissue pattern is taken out of your gut and checked for harm.

It's quality to get examined for celiac sickness earlier than attempting a gluten-unfastened weight loss program. Otherwise, it becomes difficult on your physician to inform when you have celiac sickness or now no longer.

People who don't have celiac sickness however sense they'll be touchy to gluten can attempt a strict gluten-unfastened weight loss program for some weeks to peer if their signs improve. Be certain to are looking for help from a physician or dietitian.

After some weeks, you could re-introduce meals that comprise gluten into your weight loss program and check for signs. If a gluten-unfastened weight loss program doesn't assist your signs, it's miles in all likelihood that some thing else is inflicting your digestive troubles.

SUMMARY

Gluten is a own circle of relatives of proteins this is located in positive grains. Eating it reasons dangerous results in human beings with celiac sickness and gluten sensitivity.

Why Gluten Is Bad for Some People

Most human beings can consume gluten with out experiencing aspect results.

However, human beings with gluten intolerance or celiac sickness can not tolerate it.

People with different problems like wheat hypersensitivity and non-celiac gluten sensitivity additionally regularly keep away from gluten.

Aside from an hypersensitivity, there are   predominant motives why a person might need to keep away from gluten.

CHAPTER TWO

Celiac Disease

Celiac sickness influences as much as 1% of human beings global It is an autoimmune sickness wherein the frame errors gluten as a overseas threat. To get rid of this "threat," the frame overreacts and assaults the gluten proteins.

Unfortunately, this assault additionally damages surrounding areas, together with the intestine wall. This can cause nutrient deficiencies, excessive digestive troubles and anemia, in addition to growth the danger of many dangerous diseases.

People with celiac sickness regularly enjoy sharp belly ache, diarrhea, constipation, pores and skin rashes, belly soreness, bloating, weight loss, anemia, tiredness and despair.

Interestingly, a few human beings with celiac sickness don't enjoy digestive signs. Instead, they'll enjoy different signs like fatigue, despair and anemia.

However, those signs also are common in lots of different scientific conditions, making celiac sickness hard to diagnose.

Non-Celiac Gluten Sensitivity

Non-celiac gluten sensitivity is assumed to have an effect on 0.5–13% of human beings.

People who're categorized as having non-celiac gluten sensitivity do now no longer check nice for celiac sickness or a wheat hypersensitivity. However, they nevertheless sense uncomfortable after ingesting gluten.

Symptoms of non-celiac gluten sensitivity are just like the ones of celiac sickness and consist of belly ache, bloating, adjustments in bowel motions, tiredness and eczema or a rash.

However, non-celiac gluten sensitivity is exceptionally controversial. Some specialists trust this sensitivity exists, whilst others trust it's miles all in human being's heads.

For example, one examine examined this idea on 35 human beings with non-celiac gluten sensitivity. Scientists gave contributors each a gluten-unfastened flour and a wheat-primarily based totally flour at separate instances with out figuring out them.

They located that -thirds of human beings couldn't inform the distinction among the gluten-unfastened flour and wheat-primarily based totally flour. In fact, almost 1/2 of the contributors had worse signs after ingesting the gluten-unfastened flour.

Also, those signs can be because of different irritants like FODMAPS — short-chain carbohydrates that could purpose digestive troubles.

Nevertheless, a few proof suggests that gluten-sensitivity exists

At the give up of the day, the proof surrounding non-celiac gluten sensitivity is blended. However, in case you suppose gluten is making you uncomfortable, it's quality to allow your physician realize.

SUMMARY

Most human beings can tolerate gluten, however it reasons troubles in human beings with celiac sickness and non-celiac gluten sensitivity.

Foods to Avoid

Completely fending off gluten may be challenging.

This is due to the fact it's miles located in lots of common substances which can be introduced to meals.

These are the principle reassets of gluten in the weight loss program:

• Wheat-primarily based totally meals like wheat bran, wheat flour, spelt, durum, kamut and semolina

• Barley

• Rye

• Triticale

• Malt

• Brewer's yeast

Below are a few meals that could have substances containing gluten introduced to them:

• Bread. All wheat-primarily based totally bread.

• Pasta. All wheat-primarily based totally pasta.

• Cereals. Unless classified gluten-unfastened.

• Baked goods. Cakes, cookies, muffins, pizza, bread crumbs and pastries.

• Snack meals. Candy, muesli bars, crackers, pre-packaged comfort meals, roasted nuts, flavored chips and popcorn, pretzels.

• Sauces. Soy sauce, teriyaki sauce, hoisin sauce, marinades, salad dressings.

- Beverages. Beer, flavored alcoholic beverages.

- Other meals. Couscous, broth (until classified gluten-unfastened).

The simplest manner to keep away from gluten is to consume unprocessed, single-aspect meals. Otherwise, you have to study the meals labelsof maximum meals you buy.

Oats are clearly gluten-unfastened. However, they're regularly infected with gluten, as they is probably processed in the identical manufacturing facility as wheat-primarily based totally meals.

SUMMARY

Completely fending off gluten may be challenging, because it's located in lots of common meals. The quality manner to absolutely keep away from it's miles to consume whole, single-aspect meals.

Foods to Eat

There are masses of gluten-unfastened alternatives so as to can help you experience wholesome and scrumptious food.

The following meals are clearly gluten-unfastened:

• Meats and fish. All meats and fish, besides battered or covered meats.

• Eggs. All kinds of eggs are clearly gluten-unfastened.

• Dairy. Plain dairy merchandise, together with simple milk, simple yogurt and cheeses. However, flavored dairy merchandise may also have introduced substances that comprise gluten, so that you will want to study the meals labels.

• Fruits and veggies. All end result and veggies are clearly freed from gluten.

• Grains. Quinoa, rice, buckwheat, tapioca, sorghum, corn, millet, amaranth, arrowroot, teff and oats (if classified gluten-unfastened).

• Starches and flours. Potatoes, potato flour, corn, corn flour, chickpea flour, soy flour, almond meal/flour, coconut flour and tapioca flour.

• Nuts and seeds. All nuts and seeds.

• Spreads and oils. All vegetable oils and butter.

• Herbs and spices. All herbs and spices.

• Beverages. Most beverages, besides for beer (until classified as gluten-unfastened).

If you're ever uncertain if a meals object carries gluten, it's quality to study the meals labels.

SUMMARY

A gluten-unfastened weight loss program has masses of alternatives. This lets in you to create plenty of wholesome and scrumptious recipes.

CHAPTER THREE

Health Benefits of a Gluten-Free Diet

A gluten-unfastened weight loss program has many blessings, particularly for a person with celiac sickness.

Here are the principle blessings of a gluten-unfastened weight loss program:

May Relieve Digestive Symptoms

Most human beings attempt a gluten-unfastened weight loss program to deal with digestive troubles.

These consist of bloating, diarrhea or constipation, gas, fatigue and lots of different signs.

Studies have proven that following a gluten-unfastened weight loss program can assist ease digestive signs for human beings with celiac sickness and non-celiac gluten sensitivity.

In one examine, 215 human beings with celiac sickness accompanied a gluten-unfastened weight loss program for 6 months. The weight loss program helped appreciably lessen belly ache and the frequency of diarrhea, nausea and different signs .

Can Reduce Chronic Inflammation in Those With Celiac Disease

Inflammation is a herbal procedure that facilitates the frame deal with and heal infection.

Sometimes infection can get out of hand and ultimate weeks, months or maybe years. This is referred to as persistent infection and can cause numerous fitness troubles.

A gluten-unfastened weight loss program can assist lessen persistent infection in people with celiac sickness.

Several research have proven that a gluten-unfastened weight loss program can lessen markers of infection like antibody stages. It also can assist deal with intestine harm because of gluten-associated infection in people with celiac sickness.

People with non-celiac gluten-sensitivity may additionally have low stages of infection. However, it's now no longer absolutely clean if a gluten-unfastened weight loss program can lessen infection in those human beings.

May Boost Energy

People with celiac sickness regularly sense worn-out, slow or enjoy "mind fog".

These signs can be because of nutrient deficiencies due to harm to the intestine. For example, an iron deficiency can cause anemia, that is common in celiac sickness.

If you've got celiac sickness, switching to a gluten-unfastened weight loss program may also assist improve your electricity stages and forestall you from feeling worn-out and slow.

In a examine along with 1,031 human beings with celiac sickness, 66% of them complained of fatigue. After following a gluten-unfastened weight loss program, most effective 22% of human beings nevertheless skilled fatigue.

Can Help You Lose Weight

It's common to shed pounds whilst you begin following a gluten-unfastened weight loss program.

This is as it gets rid of many junk meals that upload undesirable energy to the weight loss program. These meals are regularly changed via way of means of fruit, vegetables and lean proteins.

However, it's critical to keep away from processed "gluten-unfastened" meals like cakes, pastries and snacks, as they could fast upload quite a few energy in your weight loss program.

Focus on ingesting masses of whole, unprocessed meals like end result, vegetables and lean proteins.

SUMMARY

A gluten-unfastened weight loss program can offer many fitness blessings, particularly for people with celiac sickness. It may also assist ease digestive signs, lessen persistent infection, improve electricity and sell weight loss.

CHAPTER FOUR

Negative Effects

Despite having plenty of fitness blessings, a gluten-unfastened weight loss program will have a few downsides.

Here are some terrible results of a gluten-unfastened weight loss program:

Risk of a Nutritional Deficiency

People who've celiac sickness are susceptible to numerous dietary deficiencies.

These consist of deficiencies in fiber, iron, calcium, nutrition B12, folate, zinc, nutrients A, D, E and K and extra.

Interestingly, research have additionally located that following a gluten-unfastened weight loss program won't assist deal with dietary deficiencies.

This is due to the fact human beings on a gluten-unfastened weight loss program appear to select extra processed meals classified as "gluten-unfastened" over nutritious meals like end result and veggies.

Moreover, many gluten-unfastened variations of meals

aren't fortified with B nutrients, together with folate.

Since fortified bread is a main supply of B nutrients, human beings on a gluten-unfastened weight loss program can be susceptible to deficiency for those nutrients. This is particularly regarding for pregnant girls with celiac sickness, as B nutrients are important for the increase of a wholesome baby.

Constipation

Constipation is a common aspect-impact on a gluten-unfastened weight loss program.

Gluten-unfastened diets do away with many famous reassets of fiber like bread, bran and different wheat-primarily based totally merchandise. Eating a fiber-wealthy weight loss program may also assist sell wholesome bowel movements.

In addition, many gluten-unfastened substitutes for wheat-primarily based totally merchandise are low in fiber. This might be any other purpose why constipation is common on a gluten-unfastened weight loss program.

If you enjoy constipation on a gluten-unfastened weight loss program, purpose to consume extra fiber-wealthy end result and veggies, together with broccoli, beans, lentils, Brussels sprouts and berries.

Cost

Following a gluten-unfastened weight loss program may be hard on a good budget.

Research suggests that gluten-unfastened meals are kind of and a 1/2 of instances extra highly-priced than their ordinary counterparts.

This is due to the fact gluten-unfastened meals value producers extra cash to make. For example, gluten-unfastened meals should by skip stricter checking out and keep away from turning into infected.

If you're on a good budget, try and consume extra whole, single-aspect meals, as they value less.

Can Make Socializing Difficult

Many social conditions revolve round meals.

This could make it hard to socialize in case you're following a gluten-unfastened weight loss program. While many eating places have gluten-unfastened alternatives, there may be nevertheless a danger of meals being infected with lines of gluten.

Sadly, research have located that kind of 21% of human beings with celiac sickness keep away from social activities which will stick with their gluten-unfastened weight loss program.

That said, you could nevertheless socialize whilst following a gluten-unfastened weight loss program. It absolutely calls for a bit greater education ahead.

For example, in case you're ingesting out, name the eating

place ahead to peer in the event that they have gluten-unfastened alternatives. If you're going to a social gathering, you can want to convey your very own meals.

SUMMARY

People who observe a gluten-unfastened weight loss program can be susceptible to dietary deficiencies and at risk of constipation. Following a gluten-unfastened weight loss program also can be pretty highly-priced and make social conditions hard.

CHAPTER FIVE

Gluten-Free Menu

Here is a pattern menu with scrumptious, gluten-unfastened food.

Feel unfastened to change meal hints consistent with your liking.

Monday

• Breakfast: Overnight chia seed pudding — 2 tbsp (28 grams) chia seeds, 1 cup (240 ml) Greek yogurt and half of tsp vanilla extract with sliced end result of your choice. Let take a seat down in a bowl or Mason jar overnight.

• Lunch: Chicken, lentil and veggie soup.

• Dinner: Steak tacos — steak, mushroom and spinach served in gluten-unfastened corn tortillas.

Tuesday

• Breakfast: Omelet with vegetables.

• Lunch: Quinoa salad with sliced tomatoes, cucumber, spinach and avocado.

• Dinner: Shrimp skewers served with a lawn salad.

Wednesday

• Breakfast: Oatmeal with 1/four cup (31 grams) of berries.

• Lunch: Tuna and boiled egg salad.

• Dinner: Chicken and broccoli stir-fry — bird and broccoli sautéed in olive oil and gluten-unfastened soy sauce or tamari. Served with a small aspect of rice.

Thursday

• Breakfast: Gluten-unfastened toast with avocado and an egg.

• Lunch: Leftovers from Wednesday's dinner.

• Dinner: Garlic and butter shrimp served with a aspect salad.

Friday

• Breakfast: Banana berry smoothie — half of medium banana, half of cup (seventy four grams) blended berries, 1/four cup (fifty nine ml) Greek yogurt and 1/four cup (fifty nine ml) milk.

• Lunch: Chicken salad wrap, the usage of in a gluten-unfastened wrap.

• Dinner: Baked salmon served with baked potatoes, broccoli, carrots and inexperienced beans.

Saturday

• Breakfast: Mushroom and zucchini frittata.

• Lunch: Leftovers from dinner.

• Dinner: Roasted bird and vegetables quinoa salad.

Sunday

- Breakfast: Two poached eggs with a slice of gluten-unfastened bread.

- Lunch: Chicken salad wearing olive oil.

- Dinner: Grilled lamb served with plenty of roasted veggies.

SUMMARY

This pattern week-lengthy menu for a person on a gluten-unfastened weight loss program gives plenty of wholesome meals alternatives which can be wealthy in nutrients.

Helpful Tips

There are many beneficial pointers that let you observe a gluten-unfastened weight loss program successfully:

• Read meals labels. Practice analyzing meals labels so that you can without difficulty discover gluten-unfastened meals.

• Tell your buddies. If your buddies realize that you're at the weight loss program, they're much more likely to select locations with gluten-unfastened alternatives whilst you consume out.

• Buy a gluten-unfastened cookbook. Doing so may also assist you be extra innovative together along with your cooking and make food extra enjoyable.

• Plan ahead. If you're visiting abroad, ensure you studies locations to consume and shop. Otherwise, plan your weight loss program round masses of whole, single-aspect meals like lean meats, veggies and fruit.

• Use separate cooking utensils. If you percentage a kitchen with buddies or own circle of relatives members, ensure you operate separate cooking and cleansing equipment. You don't need to by accident contaminate your meals with gluten from different human beings' meals.

• Bring your very own meals. If you're travelling own circle of relatives, take meals like gluten-unfastened bread and pasta with you. This manner you won't sense ignored of own circle of relatives food.

If you don't have celiac sickness or a gluten sensitivity, you won't want to observe a gluten-unfastened weight loss program. While it has many fitness blessings, it additionally limits a few in any other case wholesome meals which can be wonderful for most reliable fitness.

SUMMARY

Situations may also get up that could make it difficult to paste to a gluten-unfastened weight loss program, however the pointers above can assist.

The Bottom Line

Most human beings can consume gluten with none terrible results.

However, people with celiac sickness and gluten sensitivity want to keep away from it, as it could purpose dangerous results.

While a gluten-unfastened weight loss program is restricting, there are masses of wholesome and scrumptious alternatives.

Just ensure to consume masses of whole, single-aspect meals like end result, veggies and lean protein reassets. They will maintain your belly satisfied and sell most reliable fitness.

What's extra, a gluten-unfastened weight loss program may also offer many fitness blessings. It can ease digestive signs, lessen infection, improve electricity stages or even assist you shed pounds.

THE END